The Kratom Cure

Potent Plant for Pain, Anxiety, Addiction

Joanne Hillyer

CONTENTS

DISCLAIMER

This book is not intended as a substitute for the medical advice of physicians. The reader should regularly consult a physician in matters relating to his or her health and particularly with respect to any symptoms that may require diagnosis or medical attention.

INTRODUCTION

What is the second most widely abused drug in rural and suburban Thailand? You might be surprised the know the answer is something with which you are probably unfamiliar – kratom. What substance can be used to cure depression, alleviate pain, and wean individuals from opiate and morphine addictions? You might be even more surprised to hear the answer is the same as for the first question – kratom.

So, what is kratom? Is it a dangerous, illegal narcotic, as the Thai government decided in 1943 and as other governments have agreed? Or is it a life-saving pain reliever that also can have stimulant and anti-depressant effects? That is the question we will investigate in this book.

In the first chapter, we will ask what kratom is, investigating where kratom is found and what benefits and drawbacks come with it. We will answer the question of why kratom has become more popular in recent years despite having been around for thousands of years.

We will look at the history of kratom in the East and in the West. We will follow kratom from its origins in the distant past to its use today around the world. We will check out the science behind the effects of kratom and what makes it work the way it does. We will find out why it acts like a stimulant as well as an opiate. Then we will look at some studies that have been conducted surrounding kratom and glean information about how kratom functions (and whether or not it is dangerous) from our findings. We will then answer the question of how kratom is used and how it is sold. We will discuss what the different strains are and what effects they have. We will then move on to looking at what kratom tourism in Thailand and Southeast Asia and what that entails. We investigate the benefits and potential dangers you might face. We also will look at how the traditional use and culture of kratom has evolved in Thailand and elsewhere. We will take a fascinating look at legal issues pertaining to kratom so that you know exactly where you stand if you buy it. Finally, we will have a look at where we see kratom going in future – is it going to be hailed as a great natural remedy or will it be banned completely?

It will be a journey packed with information, so be prepared to learn a lot along the way. With that expectation in mind, let us get started.

1 WHAT IS KRATOM?

What is kratom, anyway? Perhaps you have heard the word, but are not familiar with the specifics, or maybe you have some information, or maybe you have even used kratom but are looking for a more detailed explanation of what it is and how it works. In any case, you will find your answers here in this chapter and in the following chapters.

Where Does Kratom Originate?

Kratom is the Thai word for a plant whose Latin name is Mitragyna speciosa. You can find it natively in Southeast Asia, particularly in Malaysia, Thailand, and other parts of Indochina. It is a tall plant, growing around 30 feet tall normally and reaching heights of 70 feet at its tallest. It is taller than it is wide, being only about 15 feet across at its widest. Kratom leaves are broad and oval. Biologically speaking, kratom is part of the coffee family.

It has been used by Thai laborers for thousands of years as a stimulant and as a pain reliever, as well as to relieve diarrhea. Recently, since the years 2004 and 2005, it has seen a surge of popularity among Easterners and Westerners alike. However, its history spans many years before this resurgence.

What Does Kratom Do?

Kratom has two different types of effects, depending on the dosage. We will discuss what constitutes a low dose later, but for now it suffices to say that in low doses, kratom acts as a stimulant, much like caffeine or Adderall. It increases alertness and energy and makes the user more sociable. It improves mood levels and creates a sense of euphoria. Kratom also increases sexual desire, or libido. Overall, the user of a small dose experiences an improvement of demeanor and a greater sense of focus.

1

In higher doses, which we will also define later in this book, kratom acts as a psychoactive narcotic and a sedative, much like an opiate. It creates a greater level of euphoria than in the lower doses, as well as fights pain. It subdues emotional and physical sensitivity and thereby relieves physical and even emotional pain.

Some of the negative effects of higher dosages include a fluttering heartbeat and anxiety or stress. Additionally, while lower doses might help with diarrhea, higher doses can cause painful and even dangerous constipation. Also, users of higher doses sometimes experience stomach pain, insomnia, darkening of the skin, and depression. Anorexia and dangerous weight loss can result from prolonged, heavy use of kratom as well.

The withdrawal symptoms vary from person to person, depending on their habits and other factors in their lives. Withdrawal symptoms include body pain, runny nose, achy muscles and bones, jerky limb movement, and muscle spasms. They can also include psychological symptoms like anxiety and depression, hostility, aggression, and emotional liability.

A few other adverse effects have been reported accompanying kratom use, not the least of which is addiction. In addition, kratom is said to have some psychotic effects – hallucinations, delusions, and confusion. These effects were all reported by the United States Drug Enforcement Agency in January of 2013.

You might be wondering why, with all these detrimental effects, people continue to use kratom. Firstly, these effects do not occur with every use or in every user. Secondly, the benefits of the substance might well outweigh the drawbacks. Kratom has been used for thousands of years as a stimulant to promote hard work, and also as an anti-diarrheal and pain reliever.

In the last century, however, it has become more popular and its use more widespread. Why now? Let's look deeper into that question.

Why Now?

As I have mentioned, kratom has been around for thousands of years and its medicinal uses have been well known for just as long. When we wonder why the resurgence now, we must start by looking back to the surge of the opium trade in the late nineteenth and early twentieth centuries.

In Asia specifically, the opium trade flourished during the late 1800s and early 1900s. During that time period, many individuals in Southeast Asia became addicted to opium, which created huge profits for those countries and individuals trading opium. Opium is highly addictive, which caused the trade to flourish as demand continued and increased. The governments in Asia began to profit as well, as they taxed the sale of opium. This resulted in a great deal of revenue for countries like Thailand.

It was then discovered that kratom could help ease the withdrawals from opium and thereby cure the addiction. In an effort to avoid the negative side effects of opium, save money, and become more healthful, people began turning to kratom to relieve their withdrawals and cure their addictions. This resulted in the Thai government outlawing kratom in 1943 as they attempted to control the demand for opium.

Fast forward a few decades, and we come to the modern age. According to a 2007 paper by Dr. Edward W. Boyer in the American Journal of Addictions, opiates continued to be in great demand in the West, where kratom was virtually unknown. As the gray market and online pharmacies like www.drugbuyers.com began to be shut down, prescription opiates became less available to addicts, which led the opiate-consuming population to turn to kratom.

Gill Lockwood, owner of online kratom distribution company Major Kratom, has said that the internet has been instrumental in the rise of kratom. If it had not been for the web, the word about kratom might not have gotten to the West and the distribution of kratom would have been severely limited in scope.

What is Kratom?

To pull this all together into one coherent explanation, kratom is on the rise because opiate addictions have been increasing and people want to break their habits and dependence on such prescription drugs. The internet has aided in the spread of kratom use and is helping to offer a safer, less detrimental alternative to opiates.

In the next chapter, we will look at the history of kratom.

2 THE HISTORY OF KRATOM

I have already discussed a bit of the history of kratom, but let me expand on what we already know. First, we know that kratom originated in Thailand in the distant past, sometime thousands of years ago such that it seems always to have been part of Thai culture. Particularly, it has been and continues to be prominent among the people of Thailand's Deep South.

Discovery by the West

Originally kratom was used by Thai physical laborers to ease their aches and pains. They also enjoyed the stimulant quality, which helped them to work harder. It was discovered by the West in the mid-1800s. Pieter Williem Korthals, a Dutch botanist for the East India Trading Company, wrote about the plant from which kratom is derived in 1839.

E.M. Holmes named the plant in 1895 Mitragyna speciosa, based on the word for a bishop's hat, "mitre," because the leaf shape reminded him of the bishop's headgear. Holmes noted that kratom was used as a substitute for opium in rural and poor areas of Thailand. Two years later, in 1897, H. Ridley discovered that kratom was being used to wean addicts off opium.

Later on, at the beginning of the twentieth century, a man by the name of L. Wray reported that kratom was being used through various methods – drinking, chewing, and smoking. In 1907 he sent a sample of the substance to the University of Edinburgh where a man by the last name Hooper isolated the mitragynine alkaloid, though he did not name the alkaloid at the time.

The naming of the alkaloid came later, in 1921, when Fray isolated the alkaloid again and called it mitragynine. He also isolated mitraversine from the plant Mitragyna parvifolia. This substance is sometimes used as a fake kratom, lacing real kratom with it to make a less expensive product that is sold at the same price as kratom by unscrupulous dealers.

In the year 1930, a man named I.H. Burhill studied kratom to understand more about its psychoactive nature, and he found that kratom is good for fighting diarrhea and fever as a poultice and in ointment. This was later confirmed and proven again in 1975 by Thai scientist Dr. Sangun Suwamert, though the Thai people had been aware of its usefulness for thousands of years.

Legislation Against Kratom Begins

In 1940, three more alkaloids were discovered in kratom extracts, but Thai research ground to a halt when, on August 3, 1943, the Thai government outlawed the use, growth, and possession of kratom with the Kratom Act 2486. With this government legislation came the cutting down and eradication of any and all of the Mitragyna speciosa plants that the government could find, destroying habitats and devastating landscapes.

On January 28, 1993, the Myanmar government, formerly known as Burma, legislated that kratom fell under the category of controlled narcotics in Section 30 (b) of the Narcotic Drugs and Psychotropic Substances Law of the nation. Only a year later, the Burmese Health Ministry released findings that kratom was being used to relieve withdrawals and release individuals from addictions to opiates, morphine, and heroin.

Kratom Crime in Asia

In 2001, the Thai government began to crack down again on the kratom black market and the kratom industry. In that year, the Thai Narcotics Control Board revealed that kratom was the second most widely abused dug in Thailand, with centers in rural and suburban areas. They estimated that two million people used kratom in the country that year, and that number is only growing. In 2001, Thai police seized 1,270 kilograms of kratom.

The way the government ban affects the kratom industry has negative impacts on kratom users. First, kratom is of lower quality and higher price because of the ban. Additionally, other "fake kratom" substances are used and laced into real kratom or sold themselves as "pure kratom." These substances include mitrajavine from the plant Mitragyna javanica. These fake kratom substances are often untested, so we do not know their effects or interactions with other substances. This leads to dangerous scenarios for kratom users if they fall victim to dishonest sellers.

Malaysia outlawed mitragynine in 2003, and in August of 2004 they criminalized the leaf of the plant Mitragyna speciose as well. When they banned kratom in 2003, government officials organized a four-day raid of three cities in which kratom was known to be prevalent – Terengganu, Pahang, and Kelantan. In just four days, this operation resulted in 15 arrests, 245 kilograms of kratom leaves confiscated, and more than 800 liters of "air ketum," or "kratom water" (kratom tea) seized.

In 2006 the Malaysian Deputy of Internal Security Ministry, Datuk Mohamed Johan Baharum, announced that the Malaysian Attorney General had reclassified kratom from being considered a poisonous substance to being a dangerous drug. This made kratom more illegal than before, if that were possible.

Summary of the History of Kratom

Despite being a valued natural remedy for thousands of years, the Thai government chose to ban kratom in the 1940s. It is widely believed that this was more out of a need to protect the opium industry than anything else.

Fast-forward to today and we now see that it has become a banned substance in most Southeast Asian countries.

In the next chapter, we will look at the science behind kratom.

3 THE SCIENCE BEHIND KRATOM

If you are interested in science and biology, you would be intrigued to know how kratom works. If you are not, this chapter might seem like it could go over your head, but you will find it is well-explained so that whenever a scientific term is used, it can be well-understood. You will find that reading this chapter will inform you about the biological effects of kratom so that you can discuss the pros and cons of kratom use in a more educated way.

Active Compounds in Kratom

There are two main active compounds in kratom, the first of which I have already mentioned. It was the compound named by I.H. Burhill in 1921 – mitragynine. This is the substance that many countries outlaw if they do not outlaw the entire kratom leaf itself. It is the most abundant active alkaloid in the kratom leaf. An alkaloid just means that the compound is based around nitrogen atoms.

The other active substance in kratom is 7-hydroxymitragynine. It was once said to be 13 times the strength of morphine, though this has been proven to be too high an estimate. It is much more active than its sibling, mitragynine – 30 times more active by some estimates. Therefore, though it is present in smaller concentrations in kratom extracts and leaves, it could be just as potent a factor in the effects of kratom on the human body.

Biological Receptors and Kratom

There are four main receptors with which the kratom compounds mitragynine and 7-hydroxymitragynine interact to create the effects that they do. These are the μ-opioid receptors (which I will call the mu-opioid receptors), the κ-opioid receptors (which I will denote as the kappa-opioid receptors), the δ-opioid receptors (which I will refer to as delta-opioid receptors), and the serotonin receptors. German and Malaysian researchers partnered to give evidences for the opioid receptor

7

interactions in September of 2016, and American researchers have shown the serotonin receptors also play a role in kratom's effects on the human body. I will discuss each receptor interaction in turn.

Mu-Opioid Receptors

First, let me talk about the interaction between kratom and the mu-opioid receptors. Mitragynine and 7-hydroxymitragynine are both partial agonists for the mu-opioid receptors, meaning they both activate the receptor to perform the task it exists to perform. In this case, activating the mu-opioid receptor causes analgesia (pain reduction), miosis (pupil size reduction), slightly reduced blood pressure, itching, nausea, and euphoria, as well as sedation and reduced respiration, or breathing rate. Additionally, the receptor is in some way responsible for bowel movement functioning, so that when the receptors are activated, they fight diarrhea and can cause constipation instead.

Mu-opioids are not only activated by mitragynine and 7-hydroxymitragynine but also by morphine, which is the most abundant and active mu-opioid agonist in opium. For this reason, a person feels similar effects with kratom as they do with opiates like morphine, and it is why kratom can intervene and reduce withdrawal symptoms from these traditional opiates – they are replacing the opiate alkaloids with partial agonists, reducing the negative side effects while satisfying the body's craving for mu-opioid receptor activation.

Kappa-Opioid Receptors

The kappa-opioid receptor is the next receptor I will discuss. It is vital to many functions of the body and might differ in function and distribution between genders. Compounds that trigger the kappa-opioid receptors trigger changes in nociception (the experience and perception of pain), consciousness, motor control, and mood. The adverse effects of activating the kappa-opioid receptors are that they increase the chance of addiction to whatever substance by which they are activated.

It just so happens that the alkaloids in kratom, that is, the active compounds mitragynine and 7-hydroxymitragynine, are partial agonists for the kappa-opioid receptors, meaning that they partially activate these receptors. A study in Germany in January 2014 proved this affinity. This results in a few effects. First, there is an analgesic and antinociceptive effect such that pain perception is diminished and one can thereby control one's pain level with kratom. Kratom also produces hallucinatory effects in higher doses by activating the kappa-opioid receptors. Finally, as a drawback, the interaction between kratom alkaloids and kappa-opioid receptors is responsible for the addictive quality of kratom and can cause withdrawal symptoms to pop up when kratom use is discontinued.

Delta-Opioid Receptors

Mitragynine and 7-hydroxymitragynine are both agonists of the delta-opioid receptors, and therefore they activate the receptors to various tasks. It seems that delta-opioid receptors control the experience of pain like the mu-opioid receptors, but they differ in the types of nociception that they affect. The mu-opioid receptors, when activated, diminish the experience of acute pain, such as because of a recent injury, while delta-opioid receptors control the experience of chronic pain. The delta-opioids diminish the pain that lasts months and years beyond the surgery to heal the above-mentioned injury.

Additionally, delta-opioid receptors have something to do with the respiratory effects of kratom alkaloids. A study on pregnant sheep showed that high doses of delta-opioid agonists, such as the compounds found in kratom, can cause decreased respiration so that the sheep breathed more slowly and shallowly than before they were treated with the delta-opioid activating substances. However, it was shown that it had the opposite effect in low doses. This could explain why kratom acts as a stimulant in low doses and like an opiate in higher doses.

Serotonin Receptors – 5-HT2A Receptors

In Japan in 1997, a study was released that found that mitragynine inhibits the 5-HT2A receptors. These receptors are more abundant in those individuals who have experienced depression and suicidal ideation and in those who have attempted to commit suicide. They are found throughout the central nervous system and control the creation and functioning of serotonin, which is complicit in the development of depression.

It was confirmed by an American study in Ventura, California, in January 2017 that mitragynine is an antagonist of the 5-HT2A. It therefore inhibits the functioning of the serotonin receptor, which controls serotonin production, and the researchers found that mitragynine also opens up pathways for serotonin. Because the functioning of 5-HT2A receptors is linked to depression, any antagonist can be helpful in diminishing the experience of depression and creating a greater sense of well-being. Kratom seems to act similarly to popular medications for depression called SSRIs (selective serotonin reuptake inhibitors) without as many side effects such as weight gain, and while avoiding dangerous effects like suicidal ideation.

Summary of the Science of Kratom

While kratom consists of many more than the two active compounds, mitragynine and 7-hydroxymitragynine, these two molecules are responsible for the majority of the effects that are seen as a result of kratom use. The way in which kratom eases opiate withdrawals can be linked back to the mu-opioid interaction with the two kratom alkaloids, and the way that kratom can become addictive is linked to the kappa-opioid receptors. The delta-opioid interaction can explain the way that chronic pain is reduced and the mu-opioid receptors can explain why acute pain experience is eased. Finally, the 5-HT2A serotonin receptor interaction with mitragynine can explain the antidepressant effects of kratom.

Having discussed the science behind kratom, let me now investigate some studies that have been performed and reports that have been given. This will help in determining whether kratom is dangerous or not.

4 IS KRATOM DANGEROUS?

In order to look at the evidence for and against kratom use, we need to break the facts down into more informative categories than just pros and cons. We need to weigh the benefits and drawbacks, but we also need to put all the evidence together and gain an overall picture, which requires breaking down the studies and research into smaller pieces first. To break the information down into smaller and more digestible chunks, I will look at the following categories: side effects of kratom, withdrawal and dependence development, benefits of kratom use, interactions of kratom with other substances, and kratom-cited deaths. Some of the "evidence" against kratom are myths while others stand true, so I will cover each category in turn.

Side Effects of Kratom

Kratom is not without its side effects and, like any substance, will have its own interactions with an individual's biology. Therefore, the side effects and their magnitude can differ from person to person and depend on dosage.

In June 2010, Malaysian researchers found that mice treated with mitragynine, one of the active compounds in kratom, did not respond to the changing in the position of an object, suggesting that their short-term memory was affected. This could have profound effects if it is the same case for humans, as no one wants to lose their memories or forget what happened for a period of time. However, the effect has not been tested in humans, so we cannot be sure that short-term memory is affected by kratom use in humans.

A year later, in June 2011, mitragynine was found to possibly be linked to hypothyroidism in humans. It would seem, according to this study, that mitragynine lowers the effectiveness of thyroid-activating compounds by reducing the response of the thyroid to such substances. If this is true, mitragynine and kratom could cause weight gain, increase depression, and result in myriad other symptoms that go along with hypothyroidism.

In April 2013, Malaysian scientists found that only high doses of mitragynine seemed to have adverse effects on the rats they were testing. In low and medium doses, the rats remained healthy and showed no toxic effects, but in very high doses, the rats lost weight, reduced their food intake and increased their liver weight, suggesting some toxicity in high doses. Therefore, it seems likely that overdose on kratom is possible but highly unlikely, and would occur over long periods of time rather than in a single session.

Despite an American study in early 2017 stating that the side effects outweigh the benefits of kratom, it is still unclear whether kratom disadvantages really overwhelm the advantages. Overall, the side effects of kratom are known to be more dependence and withdrawal, which I will discuss next, rather than symptoms that crop up alongside the benefits of kratom. A review in the Oncologist in August 2017 spoke to that effect. In other words, only when a person decides to stop using kratom do the negative effects tend to appear.

Dependence, Tolerance, and Withdrawal

Malaysian researchers summed up a multitude of studies and reviews in February 2013 to the effect that humans can build a tolerance to kratom and develop a dependence on the substance such that they experience withdrawal symptoms should they attempt to quit using kratom. This has been a known fact for many years, though, and yet kratom users continue to tout that the benefits outweigh the detriments. Additionally, some users have found that decreasing kratom use bit by bit reduces the withdrawal effects.

Another study by German and Malaysian scientists in June 2014 showed that individuals who had been using kratom for more than six months were extremely likely to develop at least a moderate dependence on the substance, and more than half of them found themselves with an extreme dependence on kratom. Withdrawal symptoms, according to the study, included muscle spasms and pain, insomnia, watery eyes and nose, hot flashes, fever, decreased appetite, weight loss, and diarrhea. Additionally, withdrawal affected the psychology of the individuals studied such that the patients experienced restlessness, tension, anger, sadness, and nervousness. However, if it is true that withdrawal effects decrease when kratom use is tapered instead of cutting off all at once, then these effects would be minimal in a careful reduction of kratom usage over time.

In January of 2016, Germany, Canada, and Malaysia cooperated in a study that proved that physical, bodily signs of withdrawal started 12 hours after the last dose of kratom, and anxiety and other psychological effects of withdrawal began 24 hours after the last use of kratom. Though these symptoms come on rather quickly, the study failed to state how long the symptoms lasted.

To summarize, tolerance is known to occur with kratom use such that the user needs more and more of the substance to achieve the same effect. Dependence and withdrawal symptoms are also well-known to occur. These are the most cited reasons among actual users that kratom has negative effects. However, there might exist ways to reduce the effects of tolerance, dependence, and withdrawal, in that one can use kratom less frequently or taper off his or her use in order to be free of the dependence completely.

Benefits of Kratom Use

Various benefits of kratom use have been documented. In May 2017 a study was published by British, Italian, and Malaysian scientists citing kratom as a means of breaking opiate addiction as well as for use as recreation. This study proved through scientific research that kratom is effective against the withdrawal symptoms of opiates and can help treat addiction to morphine, opium, and other dangerous drugs.

Another body of research from March 2011 in Malaysia looked at the effects on rats in a forced swim test and in a tail suspension test as well as in an open-field test. In the first two tests, which tended to result in depressive symptoms, the rats treated with mitragynine showed antidepressant tendencies as opposed to the rats that were not treated with mitragynine. The open-field test had no results worth noting, on the other hand. Thus, we can see that certain stressors can activate the antidepressant effects of mitragynine, so if you take kratom in the right circumstances, you may be able to alleviate depression.

The April 2017 American study mentioned earlier also cited antinociceptive effects of kratom use, that is, the pain-killing effects of the substance. The pain-reducing effects of kratom have been known for thousands of years, as laborers would use the substance to treat their body aches and pains. The study also found that mitragynine could suppress appetite as an anorectic substance. For those who use heavy stimulants like Vyvanse for their binge eating disorders, this lighter stimulant could be a great alternative. The study also mentioned the antidepressant effects of kratom alkaloids, which we discussed earlier.

Besides these effects, kratom is a known stimulant in small doses, allowing for greater focus and concentration. However, because of its opiate-like effects, it is not as strong of a stimulant and doesn't result in the same side effects as, for example, the ADHD drug Adderall. In other words, it can promote hard work and attention to one's activity without causing racing heartbeat or other symptoms.

The benefits of kratom use are many and varied depending on the dosage you are using. If you are looking for a light stimulant to suppress appetite and increase concentration, kratom could be a great, natural option for you. If you are looking for a more opiate-like pain-relieving effect or an antidepressant, kratom could be the remedy for you.

Interactions with Other Substances

In Worcester, Massachusetts, American researchers found a detrimental kratom interaction with modafinil in June 2008. According to the research, a middle-aged man was addicted to hydromorphone and successfully cured his addiction through the use of kratom. However, soon after using kratom to alleviate his addiction, he began to experience seizures. These seizures disappeared as soon as he discontinued the use of kratom. This indicates that users need to be careful when combining kratom with other stimulants, of which modafinil is one.

Additionally, there exists a drug concoction called Krypton of which kratom is a component. In Sweden, in May 2011, there were nine cases of Krypton overdose and death reported in one year. We will discuss these deaths and their causes in the next subsection. In the same month of May 2011, German researchers reported that mixing kratom with other substances like illegal synthetic drugs and herbal concoctions could be dangerous. It is unclear whether these reports were connected. Either way, we know that mixing kratom with other compounds can be lethal, but it remains a fact that kratom on its own has not been proven to be the cause of death in any of the cases.

In fact, in September 2016, Malaysian scientists reported that there have been no known deaths because of kratom in Asia. Rather, the researchers connected the deaths in the West that occurred in connection to kratom with the use of other substances in concoction with kratom. They suggested that kratom itself is safe, but mixing kratom with other chemicals is not, and it might not even be the mixture, but the other chemicals themselves that are the problem.

Deaths Connected to Kratom

In the United States, the Drug Enforcement Administration reported that it was aware of 15 deaths between 2014 and 2016 related to kratom. Nine of these deaths were connected to the use of Krypton, which is a concoction of kratom and a substance called O-desmethyltramadol (ODSMT for short). According to an article published in June 2017, these nine deaths were due to the overdose of the substance, ODSMT, rather than kratom.

Another report by a Denver, Colorado, news station sensationalized the death of Guy Garcia in 2014. He was said by the coroners to have died from an overdose of mitragynine. The language used in the article clearly shows a bias against kratom, and the article contained a lack of any scientific information about mitragynine and kratom.

It is true that there have been other reports of deaths involving kratom. In January 2013, in San Antonio, Texas, coroners reported the death of a 17-year-old male by mitragynine overdose. In Norway, the next December, coroners in Norway cited kratom overdose as the cause of death in another individual. In March 2015, San

Diego forensics reported a 24-year-old male dead by mitragynine overdose, finding traces of the kratom alkaloid in his blood, liver, and other organs.

One of the most sensational (and possibly least factual) of reports came from Florida in January 2016, when a woman told the press that her son died of kratom withdrawals. Specifically, he committed suicide and his mother reported kratom as the culprit.

Summary of Whether Kratom is Dangerous

What do these reports mean for the future of kratom? That is something I will look at in the final chapter of this book, but suffice it to say for now that kratom has fewer reported deaths in two years than prescription drugs have in a week in the United States. If we submit to the fact that our prescription medications are causing dozens of deaths each day, why are we trying to outlaw a substance with less than one death per month on average worldwide?

In the next chapter I will look at how to prepare kratom.

5 KRATOM PREPARATION

Like cannabis, kratom has many methods of consumption and comes in various strains. In this chapter, I will look at the methods by which you can use kratom, and then in the next chapter I will discuss the various strains.

Leaf Chewing

To use the chewing method, you take a fresh leaf of kratom and remove the stringy center vein and then simply chew the leaf. You keep the leaf in your mouth and only swallow the juices that are produced by chewing.

This is the preferred method of consumption in Southeast Asia, where kratom originates. However, there are two drawbacks to this method. First, you might not be able to find fresh kratom leaves where you are, meaning they will be dried by the time they get to you and have an unpleasant texture in your mouth. Second, even when fresh, the leaves are chewy and therefore might still be an unpleasant experience to chew.

If you are visiting a country or region in which kratom can be grown fresh, you might want to attempt this method, but if you are not from a place that has fresh kratom leaves, you will want to stick to another method.

Powdered Leaf Capsules

You often can find kratom as a powdered substance inside a capsule. To create powdered leaf capsules, the kratom leaves are dried and crushed into a powder and then equal amounts of powder are put inside each capsule.

These capsules have the advantage of being easy to ingest. They also are easier to use in terms of trying to get the right dosage and are popular in the online market.

"Toss and Wash" Powder Method

If you are the type that doesn't mind ingesting the powder itself and want to save money by avoiding the capsule production, try the "toss and wash" method. With this method, you simply "toss" some of the powder into your mouth with a spoon and immediately follow it up with a drink of some type of liquid, like water or juice.

The drawback to this method is twofold. First, you might cough up some of the powder because of the gag reflex and lose some of the substance that way. Secondly, it is a less precise way to obtain the dosage you want.

Powdered Leaf Paste/Liquid Preparation

Powdered kratom can be mixed with liquids like chocolate milk, orange juice, or water to create a drinkable ingestion method. You can make a paste out of the powder and ingest kratom that way, following it up with water. You also could mix kratom into your liquid food or beverage of choice, including yogurt and applesauce.

This has the advantage over the "toss and wash" method of not causing you to gag as easily. It still can be a less precise means of obtaining the correct dosage depending on whether you are using a scale or a spoon.

Here is a recipe for creating kratom chocolate milk:

Ingredients:

- Your dosage of kratom powder
- 8 ounces of chocolate milk (pre-mixed)

Steps:

1. Pour your kratom powder into the bottom of a drinking glass.
2. Pour in as much milk as there is powder.
3. Mix the two together until there are no lumps.
4. Pour a few more ounces of chocolate milk and stir until there are no lumps left.
5. Pour in the rest of the milk and mix.
6. Drink the mixture.
7. Make a little bit more chocolate milk and use it to catch any of the kratom powder left in the glass (optional).

Powdered Leaf Tea

Powdered kratom leaves can be turned into tea with the right method. Tea can be concentrated to make the correct dosage just a matter of sipping down a swig of liquid, or if you enjoy the taste of it, you can leave it more diluted. Below is a recipe for kratom tea:

1. Boil 1 quart of water with 2 ounces (about 8 doses) of dried or crushed kratom leaf.
2. Strain out the leaf particles and set aside the liquid you obtain.
3. Boil the leaf particles with another quart of water.
4. Strain the leaf particles out and discard.
5. Combine the two quarts of tea and boil down to one cup (8 ounces) of water. Be careful not to let it burn.

Water-Based Extract

Water-based extracts of kratom alkaloids are made using the same process no matter where they are derived. The alkaloids are extracted from the kratom plant and then dissolved in water, at which point they are ground into a finer powder and the water is evaporated. What is left is a brown residue that has a stronger alkaloid concentration than the original leaf.

One of the advantages of water-based extraction is that you can avoid the side effects of the high-potency tinctures and resin extracts. Also, you can use whole leaves to improve the potency of the extract. Typically, this method delivers a more stimulating experience than the plant material alone. In addition, the product can be dissolved in water or water-based liquids.

The disadvantages of this method are that you will usually need to mix this extract with the natural leaf in order to obtain the pain-relieving effects, and it is more expensive than the natural plant product. Additionally, while water-based extracts are labeled with 5X and 15X to indicate the potency of the extract compared to the natural leaf, many producers overestimate the potency. This can make it hard to figure out the correct dosage.

Resin

The process of obtaining the kratom plant resin is highly specialized. It involves cooking the kratom leaf concentrate at a very specific temperature, after which it is dried and must be kept at a certain temperature or below, or else it will melt.

The advantages of resin extraction include the fact that resin is a super-concentrated form of kratom alkaloids, so despite being less in mass, it is higher in potency. Additionally, it can be melted easily to be used quickly. Because there is less of it in terms of mass, it is easier to store.

The drawbacks to resin extraction as a method of preparation include that resin is much more expensive than the leaves of kratom themselves. Additionally, it must be stored carefully or it will melt, and resin tends to cause more side effects than the leaves on their own.

Tinctures

A tincture takes the kratom alkaloids and mixes them with alcohol to produce another option for kratom preparation. When production is done the right way, tinctures can be very potent as well as offer many methods of delivery, such as topical delivery. With topical delivery, you simply place a drop or two of the alcohol-alkaloid mixture on the place of pain, for example, and the alcohol will evaporate, leaving the alkaloids on the skin to sink into the place of pain or into the bloodstream.

The advantages of tinctures are that they can be stored easily and they are very flexible in their delivery methods. They can be used easily and without much trouble, unlike smoking or chewing in which the leaves must be prepared correctly to have the maximum effect.

The disadvantages to using tinctures to administer your kratom include the fact that potency is often very different among tinctures because of the method of preparation and the amount of alcohol added to the alkaloids. In general, this is one of the most expensive options, especially per potency. Additionally, tinctures do not always deliver all of the effects they are supposed to deliver.

Smoking

Kratom can be smoked, just like any other herb, but this is not the best way to experience kratom. Firstly, you would need to smoke about 20 grams to see any effect, which would cost significantly more than your other options. Additionally, there have not been any studies to the effect, but smoking often causes carcinogens to enter the lungs and the body, increasing your chances of developing cancer.

Summary of Kratom Preparation

There are many ways to consume kratom, from chewing, adding it to a milkshake or slugging it down, to smoking it. The method you choose will depend on your personal preferences.

In the next chapter, I will talk about the different strains of kratom.

6 KRATOM STRAINS

Now that we know how we might prepare kratom for use, we can find out what different types of kratom exist. The different types of kratom are called "strains" and represent different varieties of the same species of plant. Each variety has its own mixture of effects on the human body, and though the effects differ in intensity from person to person, the type of effect generally remains the same. There are three basic varieties of kratom and a few further differentiations from there.

Red, White, and Green Vein Varieties

If you are not familiar with plant terminology, the veins of a leaf are the lines extending from the stem up the center of the leaf and branching out to feed the rest of the leaf. In kratom, there are three main types of kratom plants – the red vein, the white vein, and the green vein varieties.

Red Vein Strains

The red vein type of kratom is known to have higher concentrations of 7-hydroxymitragynine than the other varieties, lowering its mitragynine to 7-hydroxymitragynine ratio. This makes the strain more sedating and a better painkiller, as well as better for opiate-withdrawal reduction. Users have reported that euphoria results from this strain, as well as a calming effect after the beginning kick of energy.

Many red vein users recommend this type of strain for beginners because of the sense of peacefulness and optimism it instills. Only the strongest of red vein varieties can be used in opiate addiction reduction.

White Vein Strains

White and green strains share the effects of being more stimulating than the red vein strains. White (and green) vein strains give a sense of energy, where the red vein strains sedate, and the white vein varieties tend to give the most euphoria of all the strains. Many people take white vein strains of kratom for concentration and focus as well as to keep up stamina and energy through a long day.

If you experience depression or gloominess, or if you feel tired and physically exhausted much of the time, the white vein varieties might be for you. Just be careful not to take it too late in the day, as you can develop insomnia that way. You can mix it with red vein strains to help mitigate the energy and bring more balance to your kratom experience.

Green Vein Strains

Green vein leaves of kratom are said to have an effect somewhere between that of red vein strains and that of white vein strains. The green vein provides a boost to energy while simultaneously fighting pain and providing clearer thinking. It essentially brightens your mood while mitigating your experience of pain.

It is popular on the social scene because it helps relieve anxiety and social phobias, that is, social anxiety, and can lift depression as well, making a night out easier to enjoy. Additionally, the boost of energy paired with the clarity of mind makes this type popular among athletes and those who do hard labor. Because it does not lead to drowsiness like most pain-fighting substances do, many people who struggle with chronic or acute pain turn to green vein kratom strains for relief.

Further Strain Differentiation

There is further differentiation of kratom varieties in that different regions of the world grow different strains of kratom. While kratom has nowhere near as many strains as cannabis, for example, it still possesses quite a few varieties, so in this section I take a look at just some of the different strains available.

Bali Strains

Bali Strains are known to be the most relaxing strains of kratom. These come from the Indonesian island of Bali, that Westerners know as a place of peace and seaside comfort, and the strain lives up to its name, according to users. It has a balanced alkaloid content, distributing its mitragynine and 7-hydroxymitragynine potency rather evenly.

It used to be that Bali Red Vein was not available in the United States and in other Western countries, but now you can find it online as a crushed powder or in capsules. Today, it is one of the most abundant and least expensive strains out there. It is helpful with pain and has a sedating effect. It can also aid in reducing opiate withdrawals rather effectively. This strain is recommended for newer users because of its calming effects.

Bali Green Vein is similar to Bali Red Vein, but with more stimulating effects than its Red Vein sibling. It has a high alkaloid level like the famous strain Maeng Da, and therefore is effective in lower doses than its sibling. The effects of Bali Green Vein are supposed to be stimulating and relaxing at the same time with a general sense of euphoria and elevated mood.

Though the name of the strain suggests it is grown in Bali, it is more common to find this strain growing in Borneo or elsewhere in Indonesia besides the island of Bali. Bali Green Vein (as well as Bali Red Vein) is generally known to be fast-acting, but it lasts a shorter time as a result. Generally, it tends to last five to six hours for a new user and around three hours for a seasoned kratom user.

Thai Strains

Thai strains are supposed to be part of the stimulating family of strains along with Maeng Da (a strain originating in a specific region in Thailand by the name of Maeng Da). Thai strains have an energizing effect on individuals, though the amount of energy that it supplies depends on the person's specific biology.

Red Thai (the popular name for red vein Thai kratom) is the most effective against pain, as it has an analgesic quality with the more concentrated amounts of 7-hydroxymitragynine. It is less sedating than the Bali Red Vein, but it still maintains a good amount of pain-killing effects. Red Thai lasts longer than the Green and White varieties of the Thai strain. The Green Thai and White Thai strains are more effective as antidepressants and against anxiety, as the mitragynine bonds with serotonin receptors to fight low mood and stress. Green Thai is also known to help increase focus.

Thai varieties are more often imported to the West from Indonesia, from the island of Borneo in particular.

Maeng Da Strains

Maeng Da means something like "Pimp's Grade" in Thai, and it is the strain of kratom that is considered to be one of the strongest strains available. In fact, you only need 80 percent of the dosage to achieve similar effects to other strains, and the effects tend to be more distinct and stronger with Maeng Da than with other strains.

Often people use Maeng Da to replace caffeine to achieve effects of uplifted mood and energy levels. The effects of this strain are shorter in lifespan but more intense than with other strains like Bali or Thai. Maeng Da, specifically the White Vein variety, is very effective at tempering pain in high doses and will heavily sedate the user as well as control anxiety. However, it is not as effective in low doses as other white vein strains, at least in terms of controlling pain.

Maeng Da is marketed as the "genetically grown" kratom strain from the "World's First Legal Kratom Plantation," which has led some to believe that Maeng Da kratom is a GMO (genetically-modified organism). However, this is not the case. Instead, "genetically grown" simply refers to the process by which the kratom leaves were grafted and forced to breed according to certain standards in order to achieve the highly potent effect the strain has today.

Malay Strains

Malay kratom strains are known for their purity and their history. They have been used medicinally for thousands of years and are unique among kratom strains in their efficacy, that is, their effectiveness in treating the symptoms they are being used to treat. Many high-quality vendors sell Malay strains, whether it be Red Vein Malay, Green Vein Malay, or White Vein Malay.

White Vein Malay is often used in place of caffeine, like certain types of Maeng Da. It creates feelings of exhilaration and energy, and has more of a stimulating effect. It is often used as a high-energy boost at the beginning of the day or at midday to help get through working hours. Red Vein Malay is good for sedating the user and giving him or her a sense of peacefulness and tranquility. It also helps with pain so it can ease a tired body into relaxation. Green Vein Malay delivers both of these benefits at once – the energy and euphoria of the White Vein Malay and the relaxation of the Red Vein Malay.

Malay strains originate in Malaysia, although the substance has been declared illegal by the Malaysian government.

Indo Strains

There are a few different varieties of Indonesian kratom strains, or Indo strains, from which to choose, such as Super Indo kratom, Premium Indo kratom, and Ultra Enhanced Indo kratom, which is also referred to as UEI kratom.

When you see the word "Super" preceding the phrase "Indo kratom," you can be confident that the growing method of the kratom selects large leaves with high concentrations of alkaloids. This creates a product that requires lower doses to achieve the same effects. "Super" products are considered more potent products because the strains they use are more potent.

When you see the word "Premium," you can tell that the product is produced and harvested in such a way that the stems are taken out of the leaves before grinding them into a powder. This also removes the low alkaloid, concentration parts of the plant, resulting in a more concentrated product. It is often considered a great beginner's product because it mixes cost-effectiveness with potency.

UEI kratom products mix concentrated powder with regular kratom powder to achieve higher potency. There are varying opinions about whether UEI products are worth the price.

Summary of Strain Information

There are other strains besides the ones mentioned and discussed above. For example, there are Vietnamese strains of Red, White, and Green Vein varieties, as well as Kali strains from a specific small island of Kalimantan. Strains specific to Borneo also exist. Each strain is slightly different in the combination of effects it has on the user, and even these combinations vary from user to user and dose to dose. When in doubt, try the smallest dose possible of something new and move up from there. In this way, you can avoid the negative side effects of the strains, if they have any on you, while still enjoying the benefits.

In the next chapter, we will deal with the culture of kratom and kratom tourism.

7 KRATOM CULTURE IN ASIA AND WESTERN TOURISM

Kratom, like any psychotropic substance that becomes popularized for its high, has its own culture. First I will discuss Thai and Southeast Asian culture surrounding kratom, and then I will turn to Western culture's view of and interaction with kratom.

Asian Culture Surrounding Kratom

The Thai people, as well as surrounding cultures, have been using kratom for its medicinal purposes for thousands of years. They have used it to prevent and treat diarrhea, vomiting, and fever as well as to encourage hard work among laborers and rural people.

In Asia, the traditional method is to chew the fresh leaves, brew them into tea, or dry them and smoke them. However, young users in Asian countries also like to mix the juice with other ingredients to make "cocktails." The added ingredients are meant to boost the effects of the kratom.

The typical 4x100 cocktail is not necessarily lethal – it should be made with leaf extract, cola containing caffeine, cough syrup containing codeine, and ice. When the government started tightening up controls on cough syrups containing codeine, users had to start turning to other substances.

A number of other ingredients, such as mosquito spray or paint may also be added to increase the effect, and this can make the concoction lethal.

Many users that were polled by the Phuket Gazette admitted that they started using kratom to fit in better socially, rather than for medicinal purposes. Some admitted that they were no longer able to stop using the substance.

It is also believed that some Muslim Asian users make use of the drug because it is not alcoholic but has a similar effect.

Western Culture Surrounding Kratom

Kratom use has only risen to significant levels fairly recently in the West, with many users using the drug for recreational purposes as well as for its analgesic effect. As the trees are native to Asia, most users in Western countries have to rely on the dried, powdered form or extracts.

Most users have their own preferred rituals when using kratom, with some making their own little tea ritual. Many users blend the kratom with coffee or fruit juice in order to mask the flavor of it.

Some users infuse it in ginger tea to offset the nausea associated with taking a larger dose.

Kratom Tourism

Many tourists like to travel to Thailand and enjoy the full moon beach parties. At such parties drugs and alcohol are freely available and the so-called "bucket drinks" have become popular. Young people party up a storm in a breathtaking setting where there are few, if any, taboos. It sounds like an amazing once-in-a-lifetime experience – one that most would not pass up.

However, it is not without its risks. A lot can happen when you throw alcohol and a bunch of unknown drugs into the mix. You never quite know what is being put into your bucket drink.

Tourists have complained of passing out and being robbed or raped. And the deaths of sisters Noemi and Audrey Belanger in 2012 may serve as a stark warning. While there was a lot of controversy surrounding their deaths, the official cause was attributed to the sisters having consumed some of these drinks laced with DEET. Mix in the sedative effects of kratom and you might have a recipe for disaster.

Should this put you off touring Thailand or Southeast Asia? Well, no it shouldn't – it should rather act as a cautionary tale. You can still enjoy the scenery, but steer clear of the bucket drinks.

Summary of Kratom Culture and Tourism

The evolution of kratom culture in Southeast Asia does point to a worrying trend – that of adding in sometimes dangerous substances in order to increase the high obtained. This increases the danger to those taking kratom on a regular basis.

Kratom tourism is also subject to dangers as you are potentially at risk of criminal attack or possibly death when consuming kratom with unknown substances.

In the next chapter, I will look at the legalities relating to kratom and how to know if you could get yourself into trouble by using it.

8 LEGALITIES OF KRATOM

Aside from the safety aspects there also are the legal aspects of being caught in possession of a banned substance. It is a good idea to check the laws where you live before you start to use kratom. In this chapter, we take a closer look at these laws and how they might apply to you.

Depending on where you live in the United States, you may be able to legally order kratom online. Kratom is banned in Indiana, Wisconsin, Vermont, and Tennessee. It is a controlled substance in Florida, and may only be used if you are over the age of 18 in Illinois. In Louisiana, it is banned for human consumption. At present, Iowa is reviewing legislation regarding kratom. It is legal in all other states for the moment, but the FDA is considering reclassifying it as a dangerous substance.

Kratom is completely banned in Thailand, Burma, Malaysia, Myanmar, and Australia. It is classified as a Schedule 1 drug in Denmark, Germany, Romania, New Zealand, and Finland.

Anti-drug laws in Thailand, Myanmar, and Burma are extremely tough on offenders, and tourists will not be given a free pass. And the conditions in prisons in these countries are not something you want to be subjected to. You could end up facing hefty fines or even time in jail if you are found in possession of kratom. While the authorities will take your past history into consideration, you would still be looking at more than a simple slap on the wrist.

For the moment, while stricter measures are being implemented, kratom is still legal in the United Kingdom, Korea, and Russia.

In order to keep yourself safe, make sure you know exactly what the legal status of kratom is both at home and in countries where you plan to holiday. It also is a good idea to check up on the status of kratom from time to time, as the laws could change. For example, in 2016 the DEA temporarily considered classifying kratom as a Schedule 1 drug, citing that it felt that there was potential for abuse. This would have effectively made it illegal to purchase kratom without proper medical authorization. The DEA did not follow through because there was a lot of backlash, but there is no telling if this might be repeated in future.

The scheduling and banning of Kratom is being considered in many different areas, so keep up to date with the trends in yours.

Summary of the Legality of Kratom

In summary, the legality of kratom is a fluid issue – in America, it is an issue that different states haven't agreed on. Be safe and check the laws that apply to your area before considering purchasing kratom.

In the next chapter, I will talk about how much kratom costs and how to get it.

9 THE COST OF KRATOM AND WHERE TO GET IT

In this chapter I deal with two very important points: where you can get kratom and how much it costs.

The cost is dependent on many variables – where you buy it from, what strain of kratom you buy, the effect you want to get, what form of it you buy, how you use it, and how much of it you use.

Where You Buy It From

Different vendors charge different prices – it's a marketplace commodity similar to others. That said, in areas where it is legal to use, you can expect to pay less than in areas where it is not.

Many legal vendors offer discounts on bulk purchases so you could end up paying less per ounce/gram if you buy a larger quantity overall.

The Strain of Kratom

I already have gone into detail about the different strains of kratom so I won't repeat it here. The more potent and popular the strain, the more you can expect to pay for it. So, for an extremely popular strain like Maeng Da, you can expect to pay a premium.

The Effect You Want to Get

Do you want to mellow out or do you want to feel more alert? At a lower dose, users report feeling alert and more able to cope with work. In order to feel the sedative benefits, you need to use a higher dose of the product.

What Form You Are Buying

You could choose loose-leafed tea or dried powder. The tea is slightly less expensive and usually weighs less than the same amount of powder. The tea may look like a better deal when you compare the volumes because you seem to be getting more. However, if you go by weight, you'll seem to be getting more with the powder.

Kratom in the U.S. and Europe is also available in capsule form. Some users prefer this, as they are not able to stand the taste of the tea. It is, however, a more expensive form of the product.

The extract is the most expensive, but it should be remembered that it is very concentrated. This means that you will be able to use a lot less of the extract than any other form.

How You Use It

You can choose to mix it into tea and drink it, or down the capsules. Both methods are fairly similar when it comes to how much you need to get effective results.

Kratom may be smoked, but this is not the method of choice for most users, as it is not the most effective way of delivery. You would have to smoke a lot more of the dried leaf than you would use in tea to get the same effect and this makes it too expensive for most.

How Much of It You Use

Naturally, the more you take with each dose and the more doses you take, the more it is going to cost you. Traditionally, workers using the fresh leaves started off chewing one to two leaves per day. Daily doses tend to increase to 7-10 leaves daily once the habit has been formed.

A typical dose will have an effect for around five to six hours so you shouldn't theoretically need more than two to three doses a day at most.

Assuming you are using a good-quality product, you will need to use around 2-4 grams to start to see an effect. If you want a truly stimulant effect, you will need around 3-5 grams. If you want to be calmly alert, 4-10 grams could either stimulate you or calm you.

If you want to start seeing the true sedative effects, you will need to take 8-15 grams. Note that 12-25 grams is the highest "safe" dose but also considered very high. Most people will not need to use this much.

When it comes to the extract, you should start with 1 gram and work your way slowly up to 5-8 grams at the very most, because the extract is a lot more concentrated.

Kratom is generally sold per ounce or per gram. You can expect to pay from around $9 per ounce, or $9 for 28 grams. Premium brands can come in at $21.99 per ounce, or $21.99 for 28 grams.

If you have a mild habit and take two doses every day at around 5 grams a dose, you would need about 70 grams, or 2.5 ounces a week. This would run you between $22 and $55 a week.

Where to Get Kratom

This depends on where you live. Kratom is sometimes stocked in health shops. The other alternative is to order it online. The plant itself only grows in Southeast Asia, so unless you live there, you are probably going to need to look locally or online for a supplier.

Summary of How to Get Kratom and Its Cost

In short, if you are lucky, kratom may be carried in a store near you. If not, you will need to source it online. The price fluctuates depending on demand, purity, and the strain you choose. You pay per ounce or per gram.

In the next chapter, I look at safety tips and warnings that you need to know when it comes to kratom.

10 SAFETY AND WARNINGS

There is no denying that kratom has the potential for abuse and that it may lead to addiction. But then, the same can be said for alcohol and certain commonly prescribed medications. In this chapter I look at how you can use kratom safely.

Using kratom safely is simple if you apply good common sense and use it in moderation. Studies in Thailand have shown that those using moderate amounts of the drug on a daily basis are still able to perform in society as normal. It is when you start to use too much, or start to combine it with other drugs, like codeine, that you set yourself up for problems down the line.

Why Do You Want to Use Kratom?

Start off by figuring out why you want to use kratom. Do you want it to help you be alert? Do you want it to help you relax more? Are you hoping it will help you deal with physical pain? Are you hoping it will dull emotional pain?

When it comes to pain of both a physical and emotional nature, what you are dealing with is simply a symptom. You can treat that symptom, but unless you also deal with the underlying issue, the pain will never actually go away. And that is where the road to addiction can start. Get help from a doctor or psychiatrist if you need it. Work on dealing with the issues that are causing your pain. In some cases, such as with arthritis, there is no viable cure and pain management is your only option.

Are you doing it just because you want to fit in? This is pretty much always a bad reason to do something. Find other ways to be one of the gang, or find a new group of friends.

Choose the Right Strain

This is where knowing what you want out of the experience is really of benefit. Different strains have very different effects, allowing you to choose the one best-suited to your needs.

Find a Reputable Source

You want to get what you pay for – you need to know that the supplier knows exactly what is in their product and that it is pure and not mixed with something else.

A less reputable supplier may try to cut the product with other herbs to reduce the overhead cost – some studies have found that there are supplements on the market marked as kratom that contain no kratom at all. In other cases, the kratom levels are cut and synthetic drugs are added to improve the effect. These drugs may be dangerous and may lead to dependence. There have been cases of death in Sweden linked to the use of kratom – not because of the kratom itself, but because of the drug it was mixed with.

Your Personality Type and Your Reaction

Some people have a naturally addictive personality type or a tendency to overdo things. If this is you, it is safer to avoid kratom. Used sensibly, the chances of getting hooked are minimal.

Your first experience with kratom should allow you to gauge whether or not you might develop problems with it. If you love it and want to do it again straight away, it might be better to stop right there. If you enjoy it, but could take it or leave it, you should be okay.

Start With the Lowest Dose

Start with a gram or two at the most and see what the effect is. That way, if you do have an adverse effect to it, the impact is minimal. Do this every time you try a different strain or new brand of kratom. If you still feel that you need more of an effect, then increase the dose slowly.

Give It Time to Work

If you have just eaten a large meal it can take as long as an hour and a half to feel the effects of kratom. You can reduce this wait time by taking it on an empty stomach or at least three hours after your last meal. This will reduce the wait time to about half an hour.

Some people make the mistake of thinking that they will see results instantly and impatiently increase the dose. Give it some time and don't make this mistake.

Adjust Your Dosage According to Your Needs

Do you want to feel sleepy? Take a higher dose. Do you want to feel more alert? Take a lower dose. Take only as much as you need.

Clear the Decks

The effects of one dose will last about six hours or so and can be unpredictable. If you need to drive a delivery van all day for example, it would not be a good idea to take a dose just before heading out. While a small dose can help you to feel more alert, it can also make you very sleepy.

Take the same precautions you would every night before going to bed – make sure the front door is locked, the stove is off, no candles are burning, etc. This will cover you in the event that you do fall asleep.

It is best to choose a time where you can sit back, relax, and enjoy the experience – get whatever work or chores you need to do done beforehand.

Use It Only Occasionally

And, in this case, not every day is an occasion! If you do use it daily, there is a chance that you may could hooked on it. If you only use it every now and again you shouldn't have much of a problem.

By being selective about when you use it, you also reduce the chances that you will develop a tolerance for it. A good rule of thumb is to take it at the very most once or twice a week.

Don't Mix it With Other Drugs

To be entirely safe, do not mix kratom with any drugs that depress the central nervous system. The two will enhance the effects of each other and this can be dangerous for you. You could actually stop breathing and die.

Don't mix kratom with stimulants like yohimbe, caffeine, or amphetamines, or you could raise your blood pressure dangerously.

Summary of Safety Tips

Like most things in life, kratom is safe if consumed in moderation and used sensibly. Do not use it before driving or operating heavy machinery and do not use it you have an addictive personality. Don't mix it with any other drugs, use small doses, and only use it occasionally.

In the final chapter I discuss the future of kratom.

11 PREDICTIONS

There is no doubt that kratom is a traditional remedy that can be extremely useful. Its value in helping people overcome opiate addiction and as an analgesic make its future rather interesting.

It would appear that, when used sensibly, it is no more dangerous than alcohol, but there certainly is a potential for abuse and other negative effects, especially when mixed with other drugs. It certainly bears further investigation by the medical community, and I do feel that there will be more studies into its effectiveness and potential uses.

As for its future legal status, I believe that a look at how marijuana has been handled in the past will give a fair indication of what the future holds for kratom. Marijuana also has proven health benefits, but these are offset by the perceived potential for abuse. It is a mood-altering substance in much the same way kratom is, and so is either illegal or highly regulated.

Will the medicinal benefits of kratom be deemed important enough for it to remain unscheduled? Sadly, I doubt it. Recent evidence points to the opposite being true. With more and more states in the U.S. contemplating banning it, and many countries already having done so, I believe that the die has been cast.

I don't think that the DEA is going to let the matter drop, and if kratom becomes a scheduled substance in America, other countries that are on the fence will follow suit.

What I do believe will happen is that its medicinal benefits will carry some weight with legislators. In the same way that medical marijuana may be prescribed in special circumstances, you might be able to get a prescription for kratom even if it is banned.

Summary of Predictions

The future of kratom seems uncertain. If we look at the developing trends, it seems as if its regulation will not stop any time soon.

Now it's time to wrap everything up and summarize what has been learned.

12 CONCLUSION

Thank you for joining me on this interesting journey. Whether you view kratom as a helpful natural herb or a drug that needs to be stamped out, you must agree that it is intriguing.

It has been relied upon for thousands of years as a natural stimulant and analgesic. Studies seem to indicate that it is second only to opiates when it comes to analgesic properties. Combine that with its usefulness in breaking opiate addiction and its mental and physical benefits and it is a pretty powerful natural cure.

However, like anything natural, it also has the potential to harm us if we abuse it. And that potential for harm is of concern. Studies have shown that, with regular use, kratom might be just as addictive as opiates. It is a very hard habit to break. And while indications are that it is lower in toxicity, the evolving culture of combining it with other mind-altering substances can be dangerous. Combined with stimulants like caffeine or speed, it could lead to a dangerous increase in blood pressure. Combined with substances that depress the central nervous system, like codeine, it could lead to respiratory arrest.

Add in the fluid state of the legality of kratom and the issue becomes more complex. Currently it is banned in several countries, or on the list of controlled substances. In America, it becomes even more complex because it has only been banned in some states. What is legal today might quickly become illegal tomorrow, and what do you do if you are no longer able to buy kratom legally once you've become accustomed to using it?

The potential medical applications of kratom are extensive, but some are concerned that isn't enough to overcome the potential danger.

FINAL WORDS

Congratulations! You have reached the end of *Kratom: Potent Plant for Pain, Anxiety, Addiction*. This book was designed to give you an in-depth review of kratom and how remarkable this naturally occurring substance truly is.

By now you should understand better what kratom is and how it is used. I'm excited about what the future holds for this fascinating plant and how research will evolve and bring to light the enormous potential of kratom. I hope my book has inspired you to keep up to date with the ever-changing world of kratom and helped change your perspective on it. Thanks for taking this journey with me.

If you enjoyed this book, please take the time to leave me a review on Amazon. I appreciate your honest feedback, and it really helps me to continue producing high-quality books. If you did like it please check out my other books! Just click on the cover images below to go directly to Amazon.

And please join my mailing list. You can go here to sign up: https://joannehillyerwrites.wixsite.com/home. You can look forward to bonus content, reader surveys, and announcements about upcoming books.

ABOUT THE AUTHOR

Joanne Hillyer has a lifelong interest in wellness, healthy eating, alternative medicine, and the outdoors. She is especially interested in using easily found tools and ingredients for improving healthy living. Born and raised in the Pacific Northwest, she enjoys the great outdoors, travel, cooking, and walking.

Made in the USA
Coppell, TX
28 January 2021